Preface :

ECMO (Extracorporeal membrane oxygenation) is a life support technique that provides temporary respiratory and/or circulatory support for patients with severe respiratory or cardiac failure. It involves using a machine that pumps and oxygenates blood outside the body, allowing the heart and lungs to rest and heal.

During ECMO, a catheter is placed into a large vein or artery, usually in the neck, groin, or chest. Blood is then removed from the body and circulated through a membrane oxygenator, which adds oxygen to the blood and removes carbon dioxide. The oxygenated blood is then returned to the body, bypassing the heart and lungs.

ECMO is typically used as a last resort for patients who have failed conventional therapies, such as mechanical ventilation or medication. It can be used for patients of all ages, from neonates to adults, and may be used for several days to weeks until the patient's underlying condition improves.

ECMO is a complex and resource-intensive therapy that requires specialized equipment, trained personnel, and close monitoring. It is associated with a number of potential complications, such as bleeding, infection, and clotting, and therefore should be used only in carefully selected patients by experienced healthcare providers.

Perfusionists play a critical role in the use of ECMO (Extracorporeal membrane oxygenation) therapy. They are specialized healthcare professionals who operate the ECMO machine and monitor the patient's blood flow, oxygenation, and other vital signs during the ECMO treatment.

During ECMO therapy, the perfusionist is responsible for setting up and managing the ECMO circuit, which includes the oxygenator, pumps, filters, and other components. They ensure that the ECMO machine is working properly and adjust the blood flow, oxygen and carbon dioxide levels as needed to maintain the patient's physiological stability.

Perfusionists also play a crucial role in managing potential complications associated with ECMO, such as bleeding, clotting, and infection. They are trained to recognize and respond quickly to any changes in the patient's condition and can adjust the ECMO circuit accordingly.

In addition to their technical responsibilities, perfusionists work closely with the ECMO team, which includes physicians, nurses, and other healthcare providers. They collaborate to develop and implement the patient's care plan, monitor the patient's response to treatment, and make recommendations for adjusting the ECMO therapy as needed.

Overall, the perfusionist plays a vital role in the use of ECMO therapy, helping to ensure safe and effective care for patients with severe respiratory or cardiac failure.

Perfusion technology is a vital component of cardiac surgery, and the role of perfusionists is crucial in ensuring patient safety and successful outcomes. By dedicating yourselves to learning more about perfusion technology, you are making a significant contribution to the field, and are demonstrating your commitment to the well-being of your patients.

I encourage you to continue your pursuit of knowledge and excellence in this field, and to stay engaged with the latest developments and best practices. By remaining curious, open-minded, and willing to learn, you can continue to grow and develop your skills as perfusionists, and make a meaningful impact in the lives of your patients.

Remember that every patient is unique, and every case presents its own challenges and opportunities. By staying focused, collaborative, and compassionate, you can help to ensure that your patients receive the highest quality of care, and achieve the best possible outcomes.

Thank you for your dedication to the field of perfusion technology, and for your commitment to improving patient care. Your efforts are truly appreciated, and I wish you all the best in your future endeavors.

TOPICS

1. History of ECMO
2. Advantages of ECMO
3. Benefits of ECMO
4. Patient selection for ECMO
5. Indications for ECMO
6. Contraindications of ECMO
7. Complications during ECMO
8. Veno-Venous ECMO
9. Veno-Arterial ECMO
10. Components of ECMO
11. ECMO circuit diagram
12. Cannula selection for ECMO
13. Motioning of patient on ECMO
14. Ultrafiltration on ECMO
15. Maintenance of ECMO circuit
16. Clinical setup & Monitoring
17. Weaning OFF ECMO
18. Cannula size selection for ECMO

1. History of ECMO

ECMO (Extracorporeal membrane oxygenation) therapy has a relatively short history, dating back to the 1970s. The first successful use of ECMO was reported in 1972 when a team of researchers at the University of California, Los Angeles (UCLA) used a pump-oxygenator device to support the circulation of a patient with acute respiratory failure.

In the following years, ECMO was used mainly as a last resort treatment for neonatal respiratory failure, with variable success rates. However, in the 1980s, improvements in technology, including the development of more efficient oxygenators and better anticoagulation management, led to improved outcomes in both neonatal and adult patients.

In the 1990s, ECMO began to be used more widely for a variety of respiratory and cardiac conditions, including acute respiratory distress syndrome (ARDS), acute myocardial infarction (AMI), and pulmonary embolism. ECMO has since become a standard treatment option in many hospitals around the world, particularly for patients with severe respiratory or cardiac failure that has failed to respond to conventional therapies.

Today, ECMO continues to evolve, with ongoing research aimed at improving patient selection, reducing complications, and expanding the use of ECMO to new indications. While ECMO remains a complex and resource-intensive therapy, it has provided a life-saving option for many patients who would have had limited or no treatment options in the past.

While ECMO remains a complex and resource-intensive therapy, it has provided a life-saving option for many patients who would have had limited or no treatment options in the past. The ongoing research aims to improve patient selection, reduce complications, and expand the use of ECMO to new indications.

Here are some of the milestones in the history of ECMO (Extracorporeal membrane oxygenation) therapy:

- 1972: First successful use of ECMO reported at the University of California, Los Angeles (UCLA) to support a patient with acute respiratory failure.
- 1975: First successful use of ECMO in a neonate reported by a team at the University of Michigan.
- 1980s: Advancements in technology, including the development of more efficient oxygenators and better anticoagulation management, led to improved outcomes in both neonatal and adult patients.
- 1985: The first randomized controlled trial of ECMO for neonatal respiratory failure showed a significant reduction in mortality.
- 1994: The first successful use of ECMO in a patient with H1N1 influenza reported in Australia, leading to increased interest in ECMO for severe respiratory failure.
- 2000s: The use of ECMO expanded to new indications, including acute myocardial infarction (AMI), pulmonary embolism, and trauma.
- 2009: The H1N1 influenza pandemic led to a surge in ECMO use, with reports of improved outcomes in some patients.
- 2011: The CESAR trial showed improved outcomes and reduced healthcare costs with ECMO compared to conventional management for severe acute respiratory distress syndrome (ARDS).
- 2018: The EOLIA trial showed improved survival with ECMO compared to conventional management for severe ARDS.
- Today: ECMO continues to be used as a life-saving therapy for patients with severe respiratory or cardiac failure, with ongoing research focused on improving patient selection, reducing complications, and expanding the use of ECMO to new indications.

Overall, these milestones demonstrate the significant impact of ECMO on critical care medicine and the ongoing evolution of this complex therapy.

The development of ECMO (Extracorporeal membrane oxygenation) therapy was the result of the collaborative efforts of several researchers and clinicians. However, two names are commonly associated with the founding of ECMO: Dr. Robert Bartlett and Dr. Robert H. "Bud" Fong.

Dr. Robert Bartlett, a surgeon at the University of Michigan, was one of the pioneers of ECMO. In 1975, he and his team successfully used ECMO to treat a newborn with respiratory failure, marking the first successful use of ECMO in a neonate. Dr. Bartlett also led the development of the first commercially available ECMO system, known as the "Michigan Mark V" ECMO circuit.

Dr. Robert H. "Bud" Fong, a pediatrician at the University of California, Los Angeles (UCLA), is also credited with playing a key role in the development of ECMO. In 1972, he and his team successfully used a pump-oxygenator device to support the circulation of a patient with acute respiratory failure, marking the first successful use of ECMO in a human.

Dr. Fong also played a key role in the development of the "Los Angeles" ECMO circuit, which was an early version of the ECMO machine.

While these two individuals are often credited as the founders of ECMO, it is important to recognize the contributions of the many researchers, engineers, and clinicians who have helped to develop and refine this life-saving therapy over the years.

2. Advantages of ECMO

ECMO (Extracorporeal membrane oxygenation) therapy is used as a life-saving treatment for patients with severe respiratory or cardiac failure that has failed to respond to conventional therapies. The therapy involves the use of a specialized machine that pumps and oxygenates the patient's blood outside of the body, allowing the lungs or heart to rest and heal.

The primary indications for ECMO include:

1. Respiratory failure: ECMO is used to support patients with severe respiratory failure due to conditions such as acute respiratory distress syndrome (ARDS), pneumonia, or influenza.
2. Cardiac failure: ECMO is used to support patients with severe cardiac failure due to conditions such as myocardial infarction, myocarditis, or cardiac arrest.
3. Extracorporeal cardiopulmonary resuscitation (ECPR): ECMO is used as a rescue therapy for patients in cardiac arrest who are unresponsive to conventional resuscitation measures.
4. Bridge to transplant: ECMO is used as a temporary support to keep patients alive while they await a lung or heart transplant.
5. Bridge to recovery: ECMO is used to support patients with reversible respiratory or cardiac failure while they recover from an acute illness or injury.

ECMO is typically used as a last resort when conventional therapies have failed and the patient's condition is life-threatening. While ECMO remains a complex and resource-intensive therapy, it has provided a life-saving option for many patients who would have had limited or no treatment options in the past.

3. Benefits of ECMO

ECMO (Extracorporeal membrane oxygenation) therapy can provide several benefits for patients with severe respiratory or cardiac failure, including:

1. Improved oxygenation and circulation: ECMO provides a temporary solution for patients with severe respiratory or cardiac failure by pumping and oxygenating the blood outside of the body, allowing the lungs or heart to rest and heal. This can improve oxygenation and circulation, reducing the risk of organ damage or failure.
2. Decreased workload for the lungs or heart: By providing temporary support, ECMO can help reduce the workload on the lungs or heart, allowing them to recover and heal.
3. Bridge to recovery or transplant: ECMO can provide patients with a bridge to recovery or transplant, giving them time to recover from an acute illness or injury or to receive a lung or heart transplant.
4. Improved survival rates: Studies have shown that ECMO can improve survival rates in patients with severe respiratory or cardiac failure when conventional therapies have failed.
5. Improved quality of life: In some cases, ECMO can help improve the quality of life for patients by providing them with a chance to recover and regain their health.

While ECMO remains a complex and resource-intensive therapy, it has provided a life-saving option for many patients who would have had limited or no treatment options in the past. The ongoing research aims to further improve outcomes and expand the use of ECMO to new indications.

4. Patient selection for ECMO

Patient selection is a crucial factor in determining the success of ECMO (Extracorporeal membrane oxygenation) therapy. ECMO is a complex and resource-intensive therapy that carries potential risks, so careful consideration is essential when selecting patients for this treatment.

The following are some of the factors that are considered when selecting patients for ECMO therapy:

1. Severity of respiratory or cardiac failure: ECMO is typically used as a last resort for patients with severe respiratory or cardiac failure that has failed to respond to conventional therapies. The severity of the patient's condition is a key factor in determining whether ECMO is appropriate.
2. Reversibility of the underlying condition: ECMO is most effective when the underlying condition causing the respiratory or cardiac failure is reversible. The ECMO therapy provides temporary support to allow the patient's lungs or heart to rest and heal, but the underlying condition must be treatable for ECMO to be successful.
3. Age and comorbidities: The patient's age and comorbidities, such as pre-existing medical conditions, are important factors in determining whether ECMO is appropriate. Older patients or those with significant comorbidities may not be good candidates for ECMO due to the potential risks associated with the therapy.
4. Timeframe: ECMO is most effective when it is initiated early in the course of the patient's illness. Delaying initiation of ECMO can decrease the chance of success.
5. Patient and family goals of care: The patient and family's goals of care should be considered when deciding whether ECMO is appropriate. ECMO is a complex and invasive therapy that carries potential risks, so the patient and family must understand the benefits and risks of the therapy and be willing to undergo the treatment.

5. Indications for ECMO

ECMO (Extracorporeal membrane oxygenation) is a form of advanced life support that can provide temporary support for patients with severe respiratory or cardiac failure. The indications for ECMO vary depending on the underlying condition and the patient's overall health.

The following are some of the indications for ECMO therapy:

1. Acute respiratory distress syndrome (ARDS): ECMO can provide respiratory support for patients with severe ARDS that is refractory to conventional mechanical ventilation.
2. Cardiogenic shock: ECMO can provide circulatory support for patients with severe cardiogenic shock that is refractory to conventional therapies, including medication and mechanical ventilation.
3. Pulmonary embolism: ECMO can provide respiratory support for patients with massive pulmonary embolism that is causing severe respiratory distress and hypoxemia.
4. Post-cardiotomy shock: ECMO can provide circulatory support for patients who have developed refractory cardiogenic shock following cardiac surgery.
5. Bridge to transplant: ECMO can be used as a bridge to transplantation for patients with end-stage cardiac or respiratory failure who are awaiting a transplant.
6. Bridge to recovery: ECMO can provide temporary support for patients with reversible respiratory or cardiac failure, allowing time for the patient's underlying condition to improve.
7. Trauma: ECMO can provide support for patients with severe trauma, such as lung contusions or traumatic cardiac arrest.

The specific indications for ECMO depend on the underlying condition and the patient's overall health. ECMO can provide temporary support, allowing time for the patient's underlying condition to improve or to facilitate further treatment.

6. Contraindications of ECMO

While ECMO (Extracorporeal membrane oxygenation) can be life-saving in certain circumstances, there are also several contraindications that must be considered before initiating ECMO therapy.
Some of the contraindications for ECMO include:

1. Advanced age: Patients who are elderly may not be good candidates for ECMO due to the increased risks of complications associated with the procedure.
2. Chronic comorbidities: Patients with chronic comorbidities, such as severe liver or kidney disease, may not be good candidates for ECMO due to the increased risk of complications associated with the procedure.
3. Irreversible neurological injury: Patients with severe, irreversible neurological injury may not be good candidates for ECMO due to the low likelihood of recovery.
4. Severe coagulopathy: Patients with severe coagulopathy may not be good candidates for ECMO due to the increased risk of bleeding complications associated with the procedure.
5. Intractable sepsis: Patients with intractable sepsis may not be good candidates for ECMO due to the increased risk of infection associated with the procedure.
6. Refractory multi-organ failure: Patients with refractory multi-organ failure may not be good candidates for ECMO due to the increased risks of complications associated with the procedure.
7. Advanced malignancy: Patients with advanced malignancy may not be good candidates for ECMO due to the low likelihood of survival and the increased risk of complications associated with the procedure.

In summary, ECMO is not appropriate for all patients, and there are several contraindications that must be considered before initiating therapy. Each patient must be carefully evaluated to determine if ECMO is an appropriate treatment option.

7. Complications during ECMO

While ECMO (Extracorporeal membrane oxygenation) can be a life-saving therapy, it is associated with a number of potential complications that must be carefully monitored and managed. Some of the possible complications of ECMO include:

1. Bleeding: Patients on ECMO are at increased risk of bleeding due to the need for anticoagulation to prevent clotting in the ECMO circuit. Bleeding can occur at the cannulation sites, at surgical sites, or in other areas of the body.
2. Infection: Patients on ECMO are at increased risk of infection due to the presence of foreign materials in the body, such as cannulas and the ECMO circuit. Infection can be local or systemic and can lead to sepsis, pneumonia, or other serious complications.
3. Hemolysis: The mechanical forces exerted by the ECMO pump can cause damage to red blood cells, leading to hemolysis (breakdown of red blood cells). This can cause anemia and other complications.
4. Clotting: The ECMO circuit can become clogged with clots, which can lead to decreased flow and oxygenation. Patients on ECMO require careful monitoring of their anticoagulation status to prevent clotting in the circuit.
5. Air embolism: Air can enter the ECMO circuit, which can cause an air embolism if it enters the patient's bloodstream. This can lead to serious complications, including stroke or cardiac arrest.
6. Pump failure: The ECMO pump can malfunction or fail, which can lead to decreased oxygenation and circulation. Rapid detection and correction of pump failure is critical to prevent serious complications.
7. Organ failure: ECMO is often used in patients with severe respiratory or cardiac failure, and these patients are at increased risk of developing multi-organ failure. Careful monitoring and management of other organ systems is critical to prevent complications.

8. Veno-Venous ECMO

Veno-venous ECMO (VV-ECMO) is a type of ECMO that provides respiratory support by removing blood from a patient's venous system, oxygenating it outside the body, and returning it to the patient's circulation. VV-ECMO is used in patients with severe respiratory failure, such as acute respiratory distress syndrome (ARDS) or severe pneumonia, when conventional mechanical ventilation is unable to provide sufficient oxygenation.

During VV-ECMO, a cannula is inserted into a large vein in the neck or groin and is advanced into the right atrium of the heart. Blood is then withdrawn from the patient, pumped through an oxygenator that removes carbon dioxide and adds oxygen, and returned to the patient's circulation via another cannula placed in another vein. This creates an extracorporeal circuit that bypasses the lungs, providing oxygenated blood directly to the body.

VV-ECMO is typically used as a temporary therapy to allow the lungs to heal and recover from the underlying injury or illness. The duration of VV-ECMO therapy varies depending on the individual patient's condition and response to therapy, but it is typically used for several days to weeks.

While VV-ECMO can be life-saving in patients with severe respiratory failure, it is associated with several potential complications, including bleeding, infection, hemolysis, clotting, air embolism, pump failure, and organ failure. Close monitoring and management of these potential complications is critical to ensure the best possible outcomes for patients on VV-ECMO.
Important :

Veno-VenousECMO is the preferred method in Pediatric and adult ECMO, whenever circulatory asist is not needed.

Oxygenation may not be as good as Veno-venous ECMO

Veno-venous ECMO (VV-ECMO) offers several advantages over other forms of respiratory support in patients with severe respiratory failure, including:

1. Improved oxygenation: VV-ECMO provides a highly effective means of oxygenating the blood by bypassing the lungs and delivering oxygen directly to the body. This can be especially important in patients with severe respiratory failure who are unable to maintain adequate oxygenation with conventional mechanical ventilation.
2. Reduced ventilator-induced lung injury: Conventional mechanical ventilation can cause lung injury, particularly in patients with severe respiratory failure who require high levels of oxygenation and ventilation. VV-ECMO allows the lungs to rest and heal, reducing the risk of further lung injury and potentially improving outcomes.
3. Improved survival: VV-ECMO has been shown to improve survival in patients with severe respiratory failure who are at high risk of mortality with conventional mechanical ventilation.
4. Improved quality of life: VV-ECMO may allow patients with severe respiratory failure to avoid intubation and mechanical ventilation, which can be uncomfortable and distressing. This can improve quality of life and reduce the risk of complications associated with prolonged mechanical ventilation.
5. Ability to bridge to lung transplantation: VV-ECMO can be used to stabilize patients with severe respiratory failure who are awaiting lung transplantation, allowing them to survive until a suitable donor organ becomes available.

While VV-ECMO offers several advantages in the management of severe respiratory failure, it is important to note that the therapy is associated with several potential complications, including bleeding, infection, hemolysis, clotting, air embolism, pump failure, and organ failure. Close monitoring and management of these potential complications is critical to ensure the best possible outcomes for patients on VV-ECMO.

.

9. Veno-Arterial ECMO

Veno-arterial ECMO (Extracorporeal Membrane Oxygenation) is a life support system that provides temporary support for the heart and lungs when they are unable to function properly. It is used as a last resort when all other medical interventions have failed and the patient is at risk of dying.

Veno-arterial ECMO works by pumping blood out of the body through a tube called a cannula, which is placed in a large vein (usually the femoral vein) and then through an oxygenator where it is oxygenated and carbon dioxide is removed. The oxygenated blood is then returned to the body through another cannula, which is placed in a large artery (usually the carotid or femoral artery). This process bypasses the heart and lungs, allowing them to rest and heal while the ECMO system takes over their functions.

Veno-arterial ECMO is typically used in patients who have suffered a severe cardiac or respiratory failure, such as in cases of cardiogenic shock, myocarditis, or acute respiratory distress syndrome (ARDS). It is a highly invasive and complex procedure that requires specialized training and expertise to perform.

While veno-arterial ECMO can be life-saving in some cases, it also carries risks and potential complications, including bleeding, infections, clotting, and damage to the blood vessels.

The decision to use ECMO is made on a case-by-case basis by a multidisciplinary team of healthcare professionals, taking into consideration the patient's overall health status and the potential benefits and risks of the procedure.

.

Important :
Veno-Arterial ECMO is mainly used in patients with Heart failure

It is used as cardiopulmonary bypass to give rest to the Heart.

Veno-arterial ECMO (Extracorporeal Membrane Oxygenation) provides several advantages in critical care situations where the heart and lungs are unable to function properly.
Here are some of the main advantages of veno-arterial ECMO:

1. Provides immediate and effective support: Veno-arterial ECMO provides immediate and effective support to the heart and lungs, allowing them to rest and heal while the ECMO system takes over their functions. This can be life-saving in critical situations where time is of the essence.
2. Increases oxygenation and blood flow: By bypassing the heart and lungs, veno-arterial ECMO provides increased oxygenation and blood flow to the body, which can improve organ function and prevent organ damage.
3. Allows for medical interventions: While the heart and lungs are resting, medical interventions such as medication, mechanical ventilation, or cardiac catheterization can be performed, which may be difficult or impossible in the presence of severe heart or lung failure.
4. Can be used as a bridge to recovery or transplant: Veno-arterial ECMO can be used as a bridge to recovery, allowing time for the heart or lungs to heal and regain function. It can also be used as a bridge to transplant, providing temporary support until a suitable donor organ becomes available.
5. Offers better survival rates: Veno-arterial ECMO has been shown to improve survival rates in certain critical care situations, such as cardiogenic shock or severe respiratory failure, especially when used in specialized centers with experienced staff.

It's important to note that veno-arterial ECMO is a highly invasive and complex procedure that carries significant risks and potential complications. The decision to use ECMO is made on a case-by-case basis by a multidisciplinary team of healthcare professionals, taking into consideration the patient's overall health status and the potential benefits and risks of the procedure.

10. Components of ECMO

An ECMO (Extracorporeal Membrane Oxygenation) circuit is a complex system that provides temporary support for the heart and lungs by bypassing them and providing oxygenated blood to the body. The ECMO circuit typically consists of the following components:

1. Cannulae: The ECMO circuit begins with two cannulae, which are large tubes that are placed into the blood vessels to draw blood out of the body and return it after it has been oxygenated. One cannula is typically placed in a large vein (usually the femoral vein), and the other cannula is placed in a large artery (usually the carotid or femoral artery).
2. Pump: The blood is then pumped out of the body by a mechanical pump, which helps to maintain blood flow and pressure. The pump is typically an external device that is connected to the cannulae.
3. Oxygenator: The blood is then passed through an oxygenator, which adds oxygen to the blood and removes carbon dioxide. The oxygenator is a membrane that allows oxygen and carbon dioxide to pass through it while keeping the blood separate.
4. Heat exchanger: The blood is then passed through a heat exchanger, which helps to regulate the temperature of the blood before it is returned to the body.
5. Pressure monitors and alarms: Throughout the ECMO circuit, pressure monitors and alarms are used to ensure that the system is working properly and to alert healthcare professionals if there is any problem.
6. Circuit tubing: The circuit tubing connects all of the components of the ECMO circuit and ensures that the blood flows smoothly through the system.

The ECMO circuit is typically managed by a specialized team of healthcare professionals, including perfusionists, intensive care physicians, and nurses, who monitor the patient closely to ensure that the system is working properly and to manage any potential complications.

11. ECMO circuit diagram

Here's a diagram of a typical ECMO (Extracorporeal Membrane Oxygenation) circuit:

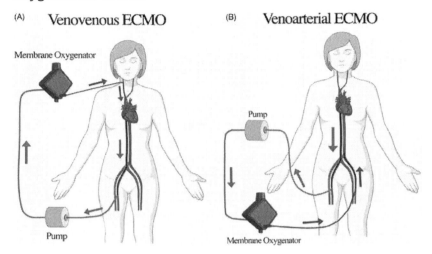

(A) Venovenous ECMO

(B) Venoarterial ECMO

Membrane Oxygenator

Pump

Pump

Membrane Oxygenator

In this diagram, the ECMO circuit begins with two cannulae, one placed in a large vein and one in a large artery. Blood is drawn out of the body through the venous cannula, passed through the oxygenator, where it is oxygenated and carbon dioxide is removed, and then returned to the body through the arterial cannula.

The oxygenator consists of a blood membrane and a gas membrane that allow oxygen and carbon dioxide to pass through them while keeping the blood and gas separate.

The blood is pumped through the circuit by a mechanical pump, which helps to maintain blood flow and pressure. Pressure monitors are used throughout the circuit to ensure that the system is working properly and to alert healthcare professionals if there is any problem.

It's important to note that this is just a general diagram and the specific components and configuration of the ECMO circuit may vary depending on the patient's individual needs and the healthcare facility's protocols.

12. Cannula selection for ECMO

The size of cannulae for ECMO (Extracorporeal Membrane Oxygenation) patients is an important consideration as it affects blood flow and overall ECMO performance.

The size of cannulae is determined by several factors, including the patient's body size, the purpose of ECMO, and the anticipated duration of ECMO support.

In general, larger cannulae allow for higher blood flow rates and better oxygenation, but they also increase the risk of complications such as bleeding and infection. Smaller cannulae have a lower risk of complications but may not provide adequate blood flow for larger patients or those with more severe respiratory or cardiac failure.

Here are some general guidelines for selecting the size of cannulae for ECMO patients:

1. Venous cannula: The size of the venous cannula for venovenous ECMO should be based on the patient's body surface area (BSA) or weight. For patients with a BSA of less than 1.5 m2, a 15-19 Fr cannula is usually sufficient, while patients with a BSA of greater than 1.5 m2 may require a 21-25 Fr cannula. For venoarterial ECMO, the venous cannula should be selected based on the same principles, but larger sizes may be required to achieve adequate blood flow.
2. Arterial cannula: The size of the arterial cannula for venoarterial ECMO is usually selected based on the size of the patient's artery. A common rule of thumb is to select a cannula that is approximately 70% of the size of the artery. For example, a patient with a 20 mm artery would require a 14 Fr cannula.
3. Double-lumen cannula: Double-lumen cannulae are often used for venovenous ECMO and provide both venous drainage and oxygenated blood return through a single cannula. The size of the cannula should be based on the patient's body size and the anticipated blood flow rates..

Cannulation sites for ECMO (Extracorporeal Membrane Oxygenation) depend on the type of ECMO support required and the individual patient's anatomy and condition.

Here are some general guidelines for cannulation sites in ECMO:

1. Venous cannulation: Venous cannulation is usually performed in a large vein, such as the internal jugular, femoral, or subclavian vein. The choice of vein depends on the patient's anatomy and the ECMO support required. The femoral vein is often preferred for venovenous ECMO, while the internal jugular vein is often used for venoarterial ECMO.
2. Arterial cannulation: Arterial cannulation is usually performed in an artery, such as the femoral or carotid artery. The choice of artery depends on the patient's anatomy and the ECMO support required. The femoral artery is often preferred for venoarterial ECMO, while the radial artery may be used for patients who require only partial support.
3. Double-lumen cannulation: Double-lumen cannulae are often used for venovenous ECMO and provide both venous drainage and oxygenated blood return through a single cannula. The cannula is usually inserted into the internal jugular vein, although other sites may be used depending on the patient's anatomy.
4. Alternative sites: In some cases, alternative cannulation sites may be used, such as the axillary vein or artery or the external iliac vein or artery. These sites may be used when the traditional sites are not accessible or when a specific configuration of the ECMO circuit is required.

In summary, the choice of cannulation sites for ECMO depends on the type of support required and the individual patient's anatomy and condition. The choice of cannulation sites should be made by an experienced ECMO team, and cannulation should be performed under sterile conditions and with appropriate imaging guidance to ensure proper placement.

13. Motioning of patient on ECMO

Patients on ECMO (Extracorporeal Membrane Oxygenation) require intensive monitoring to ensure their safety and optimize their care. Here are some of the key aspects of patient monitoring on ECMO:

1. Vital signs: Vital signs, including heart rate, blood pressure, respiratory rate, and temperature, should be monitored frequently to assess the patient's hemodynamic stability and overall clinical status. Continuous monitoring of oxygen saturation is also essential.

2. Blood gases: Arterial and venous blood gases should be monitored frequently to assess oxygenation, ventilation, and acid-base status. This information is used to adjust ventilator settings and ECMO flow rates as needed.

3. ECMO circuit: The ECMO circuit should be monitored continuously to ensure proper function and prevent complications. Blood flow rates, pressures, and oxygen saturation should be monitored at multiple points along the circuit, and alarms should be set to alert the care team to any abnormalities.

4. Anticoagulation: Patients on ECMO require anticoagulation to prevent thrombosis within the circuit. Coagulation parameters, including activated clotting time (ACT) or activated partial thromboplastin time (aPTT), should be monitored frequently to ensure that the patient is receiving the appropriate dose of anticoagulant medication.

5. Neurologic monitoring: Patients on ECMO are at risk for neurologic complications, including stroke and seizures. Neurologic monitoring, including frequent neurologic exams and monitoring of intracranial pressure (ICP) and cerebral perfusion pressure (CPP), may be necessary to detect and manage these complications.

6. Imaging: Imaging studies, including chest X-rays and echocardiography, may be used to monitor the patient's lung function, cardiac function, and ECMO circuit placement and function.

Patients on ECMO (Extracorporeal Membrane Oxygenation) require close monitoring of vital signs to ensure their safety and optimize their care.

Here are some of the vital signs that should be monitored for patients on ECMO:

1. Heart rate: Heart rate should be monitored continuously to assess the patient's cardiac function and hemodynamic stability. Changes in heart rate may indicate changes in the patient's clinical status, and should be evaluated promptly.
2. Blood pressure: Blood pressure should be monitored frequently to assess the patient's perfusion and hemodynamic stability. In patients on venoarterial ECMO, blood pressure is an important indicator of the adequacy of ECMO support.
3. Respiratory rate: Respiratory rate should be monitored frequently to assess the patient's ventilation and oxygenation status. Changes in respiratory rate may indicate changes in the patient's clinical status, and should be evaluated promptly.
4. Oxygen saturation: Oxygen saturation should be monitored continuously to assess the patient's oxygenation status. In patients on ECMO, oxygen saturation may be measured at multiple points along the circuit, including the arterial and venous lines and the oxygenator.
5. Temperature: Temperature should be monitored frequently to assess the patient's metabolic status and detect fever or hypothermia. Changes in temperature may indicate changes in the patient's clinical status, and should be evaluated promptly.
6. Urine output: Urine output should be monitored frequently to assess the patient's renal function and hydration status. Changes in urine output may indicate changes in the patient's clinical status, and should be evaluated promptly.

ECMO requires frequent and comprehensive assessments of heart rate, blood pressure, respiratory rate, oxygen saturation, temperature, and urine output.

Heart Rate

The patient's heart rate on ECMO (Extracorporeal Membrane Oxygenation) is an important vital sign that requires close monitoring.

In patients on venoarterial ECMO, the heart rate is an important indicator of cardiac function and hemodynamic stability.

Here are some key points regarding heart rate monitoring for patients on ECMO:

1. Continuous monitoring: Heart rate should be monitored continuously using a bedside monitor or electrocardiogram (ECG) to assess the patient's cardiac function and detect any changes in heart rate.
2. Baseline heart rate: The patient's baseline heart rate should be established before ECMO initiation, and any changes in heart rate should be compared to the baseline rate.
3. Tachycardia: Tachycardia (a heart rate above the normal range) may be a sign of inadequate ECMO support or cardiac dysfunction. In patients on venoarterial ECMO, tachycardia may indicate that the patient is relying on their own heart function to maintain blood flow, which can put additional strain on the heart.
4. Bradycardia: Bradycardia (a heart rate below the normal range) may be a sign of inadequate ECMO support or hypoxemia. In patients on venoarterial ECMO, bradycardia may indicate that the heart is not receiving enough oxygenated blood from the ECMO circuit.
5. Management of heart rate changes: Any changes in heart rate should be evaluated promptly. In some cases, adjustments to the ECMO flow rate, ventilation settings, or medications may be necessary to optimize the patient's hemodynamic status and heart rate.

The ECMO care team should work together to ensure that the patient receives appropriate monitoring and care.

Blood Pressure

Monitoring the blood pressure of a patient on ECMO (Extracorporeal Membrane Oxygenation) is crucial for ensuring the success of the treatment.

Blood pressure is one of the vital signs that need to be closely monitored in patients on ECMO. The ECMO circuit can affect blood pressure in several ways, including by increasing the resistance to blood flow, altering the balance of fluids in the body, and affecting the function of the heart. Therefore, it is essential to monitor blood pressure frequently and adjust the ECMO settings accordingly.

Non-invasive blood pressure monitoring methods, such as the use of a sphygmomanometer (blood pressure cuff) or an arterial line, can be used to monitor blood pressure in patients on ECMO. Invasive blood pressure monitoring is typically more accurate and reliable than non-invasive methods and involves placing a catheter in an artery to directly measure blood pressure. However, invasive monitoring also carries a higher risk of complications, such as bleeding, infection, and blood vessel damage.

The target blood pressure range for patients on ECMO varies depending on the underlying condition and the ECMO configuration. In general, the goal is to maintain a mean arterial pressure (MAP) of at least 60 mmHg to ensure adequate organ perfusion. However, higher or lower targets may be necessary in some cases. It is important to closely monitor the patient's blood pressure and adjust the ECMO settings and medications as needed to maintain the target range.

Several factors can cause changes in the blood pressure of a patient on ECMO. These factors include:

1. ECMO circuit settings: The ECMO circuit settings, such as the blood flow rate, oxygen flow rate, and circuit pressure, can affect blood pressure. For example, increasing the blood flow rate can increase blood pressure, while decreasing it can lower blood pressure.
2. Fluid balance: ECMO can affect fluid balance in the body, which can in turn affect blood pressure. Patients on ECMO may require fluids to maintain blood volume, but excessive fluid administration can lead to fluid overload and high blood pressure.
3. Medications: Some medications used in patients on ECMO, such as vasopressors and inotropes, can affect blood pressure. These medications can increase blood pressure by constricting blood vessels or increasing the heart's contractility.
4. Underlying condition: The underlying condition that necessitated ECMO, such as respiratory or cardiac failure, can also affect blood pressure. For example, low blood pressure can be a symptom of severe heart failure, while high blood pressure can be a symptom of pulmonary hypertension.
5. Patient-specific factors: The patient's age, overall health, and individual response to ECMO can also affect blood pressure. For example, older patients may be more prone to low blood pressure, while patients with a history of hypertension may be more prone to high blood pressure.

It is important to monitor blood pressure closely in patients on ECMO and adjust the ECMO settings and medications as needed to maintain a target range. Regular assessment of the patient's fluid status, medication regimen, and underlying condition can also help identify and manage factors that may be contributing to changes in blood pressure.

Respiratory Rate

Respiratory rate is one of the vital signs that need to be closely monitored in patients on ECMO (Extracorporeal Membrane Oxygenation).

Respiratory rate is the number of breaths taken per minute and is an indicator of how well the lungs are functioning. ECMO provides respiratory support to patients with severe respiratory failure, so their respiratory rate may be lower than normal. However, it is essential to monitor the patient's respiratory rate closely to ensure adequate oxygenation and ventilation.

Monitoring the patient's respiratory rate can be done non-invasively using a respiratory monitor, which measures the number of breaths per minute. The target respiratory rate for patients on ECMO varies depending on the underlying condition and the ECMO configuration. In general, the goal is to maintain a respiratory rate that ensures adequate oxygenation and ventilation while avoiding overventilation, which can lead to lung injury.

In addition to monitoring respiratory rate, other parameters such as oxygen saturation, carbon dioxide levels, and lung compliance should also be closely monitored in patients on ECMO. These parameters can help guide adjustments in the ECMO settings and mechanical ventilation to ensure optimal lung function and patient outcomes.

Close monitoring of the patient's condition and regular assessments by a multidisciplinary team, including critical care physicians, respiratory therapists, and ECMO specialists, is essential to manage respiratory rate and ensure successful ECMO therapy.

Oxygen Saturation

Oxygen saturation is the percentage of hemoglobin in the blood that is bound to oxygen, and it is an indicator of how well the lungs are oxygenating the blood. In patients on ECMO, oxygen saturation is typically monitored using pulse oximetry, which measures the oxygen saturation level in the blood noninvasively.

The target oxygen saturation for patients on ECMO varies depending on the underlying condition and the ECMO configuration. In general, the goal is to maintain an oxygen saturation level that ensures adequate tissue oxygenation while avoiding excessive oxygen exposure, which can lead to oxygen toxicity.

Monitoring the patient's oxygen saturation level is critical to ensure adequate oxygenation and adjust the ECMO settings as needed. If the oxygen saturation is too low, the ECMO machine may need to be adjusted to increase oxygen flow or blood flow rates. If the oxygen saturation is too high, the ECMO machine may need to be adjusted to decrease oxygen flow or blood flow rates.

In addition to monitoring oxygen saturation, other parameters such as respiratory rate, carbon dioxide levels, and lung compliance should also be closely monitored in patients on ECMO. These parameters can help guide adjustments in the ECMO settings and mechanical ventilation to ensure optimal lung function and patient outcomes.

Close monitoring of the patient's condition and regular assessments by a multidisciplinary team, including critical care physicians, respiratory therapists, and ECMO specialists, is essential to manage oxygen saturation and ensure successful ECMO therapy.

Temperature

Maintaining a stable body temperature is essential for patients on ECMO to minimize complications such as bleeding, infections, and hypothermia. Hypothermia, or low body temperature, can cause a decrease in cardiac output, increase the risk of bleeding, and impair coagulation. Hyperthermia, or high body temperature, can lead to increased metabolic demands, oxygen consumption, and the risk of infection.

Temperature management in patients on ECMO can be challenging due to the invasive nature of the therapy and the use of the ECMO circuit, which can affect heat exchange.

Temperature monitoring is typically done using a rectal, esophageal, or bladder thermometer to ensure accurate temperature readings. The target temperature for patients on ECMO varies depending on the underlying condition and the ECMO configuration, but a target range of 36-38°C is commonly used during ECMO.

To maintain a stable body temperature, patients on ECMO may require external warming or cooling measures, such as warming blankets, cooling pads, or an ECMO circuit heater-cooler unit. It is important to closely monitor the patient's body temperature and adjust the temperature management strategy as needed to prevent hypothermia or hyperthermia.

In addition to temperature monitoring, other parameters such as oxygen saturation, respiratory rate, and blood pressure should also be closely monitored in patients on ECMO. Close monitoring of the patient's condition and regular assessments by a multidisciplinary team, including critical care physicians, respiratory therapists, and ECMO specialists, is essential to manage body temperature and ensure successful ECMO therapy.

Urine Output

Urine output is a valuable indicator of renal function and fluid balance in patients on ECMO.

Decreased urine output can indicate renal dysfunction or hypovolemia, while increased urine output can indicate fluid overload or diuresis. The target urine output for patients on ECMO varies depending on the underlying condition and the ECMO configuration. However, a urine output of at least 0.5-1 mL/kg/hour is generally considered adequate for most patients.

To manage urine output in patients on ECMO, the following strategies can be employed:

1. Maintain adequate fluid balance: Adequate fluid administration is essential to maintain optimal renal function and urine output in patients on ECMO. The fluid balance should be closely monitored, and adjustments made to fluid administration as necessary to ensure adequate urine output without causing fluid overload.
2. Adjust ECMO settings: ECMO settings such as blood flow rate, sweep gas flow rate, and oxygen flow rate can affect renal perfusion and urine output. Adjusting these settings as needed may help maintain adequate urine output.
3. Use diuretics: Diuretics can be used to increase urine output in patients with fluid overload or decreased urine output. However, diuretics should be used with caution in patients on ECMO as they can cause electrolyte imbalances and affect ECMO circuit function.
4. Monitor medications: Several medications can affect renal function and urine output, such as vasopressors, inotropes, and sedatives. Monitoring medication dosages and adjusting them as necessary may help maintain optimal urine output.

Blood Gases on ECMO

Managing blood gases is a critical aspect of ECMO (Extracorporeal Membrane Oxygenation) therapy.
Here are some tips for managing patient blood gases on ECMO:

1. Monitor arterial blood gases (ABGs): Regular monitoring of ABGs is essential for managing patient blood gases on ECMO. ABG samples should be taken frequently to monitor the patient's oxygenation status and acid-base balance.
2. Adjust ECMO flow rates: The ECMO flow rate affects the patient's oxygenation and ventilation, and it should be adjusted based on the patient's ABG results. The medical team should aim to achieve target oxygenation and ventilation goals while avoiding excessive blood flow rates that can lead to hemolysis or clotting.
3. Adjust ventilator settings: The ventilator settings should be adjusted to optimize lung recruitment and prevent barotrauma. The goal is to achieve adequate oxygenation and ventilation while minimizing ventilator-induced lung injury.
4. Manage sweep gas flow rates: The sweep gas flow rate affects the removal of carbon dioxide (CO_2) from the patient's blood. The sweep gas flow rate should be adjusted to maintain target CO_2 levels while avoiding excessive gas exchange that can lead to hyperventilation or respiratory alkalosis.
5. Adjust oxygenation and ventilation goals: The oxygenation and ventilation goals should be adjusted based on the patient's condition, disease progression, and ABG results. The medical team should aim to achieve adequate oxygenation and ventilation while avoiding complications such as hyperoxia or acid-base imbalances.
6. Manage blood transfusions: Blood transfusions can affect the patient's oxygenation status and acid-base balance. The medical team should carefully monitor the patient's hemoglobin levels and adjust blood transfusions as needed to maintain adequate oxygenation and prevent complications such as volume overload.

The goal of ECMO therapy is to maintain adequate oxygenation. The target oxygen saturation (SaO2) depends on the patient's condition, but it typically ranges from 88% to 95%. The partial pressure of oxygen (PaO2) should be maintained at a level that achieves the target SaO2, while avoiding hyperoxia. PaO2 levels between 50-80 mmHg are usually targeted.

The partial pressure of carbon dioxide (PaCO2) should be maintained within the normal range (35-45 mmHg) to prevent acid-base imbalances.

The pH level on ECMO should be maintained within the normal range (7.35-7.45) to prevent acid-base imbalances. The medical team should monitor the patient's acid-base balance and adjust ventilation and ECMO settings as needed to maintain a normal pH level.

The hemoglobin level on ECMO should be maintained within the normal range (12-15 g/dL) to ensure adequate oxygen carrying capacity. The medical team should monitor the patient's hemoglobin level and adjust blood transfusions as needed to maintain a normal hemoglobin level.

Electrolytes :

1. Electrolyte replacement may be necessary to maintain normal electrolyte levels during ECMO therapy. The medical team may use various electrolyte solutions, such as saline, potassium chloride, calcium gluconate, and magnesium sulfate, to replace electrolytes as needed. The concentration and volume of these solutions may vary depending on the patient's clinical condition and electrolyte levels.
2. Alkalosis and acidosis: ECMO therapy can affect the patient's acid-base balance, leading to alkalosis or acidosis. The medical team may adjust the patient's ventilation or use bicarbonate to correct acid-base imbalances.
3. Risks: Electrolyte imbalances can have serious consequences for patients on ECMO, including arrhythmias, seizures, and cardiac arrest.

Anticoagulation on ECMO

Anticoagulation is a critical aspect of ECMO (Extracorporeal Membrane Oxygenation) therapy. ECMO involves the circulation of the patient's blood outside the body, which increases the risk of blood clots forming in the ECMO circuit and the patient's bloodstream.

 Anticoagulation is necessary to prevent clot formation and maintain the patency of the ECMO circuit, but it also increases the risk of bleeding complications.

Here are some key considerations for anticoagulation on ECMO:

• Anticoagulation strategies: Unfractionated heparin is the most commonly used anticoagulant for ECMO therapy. Heparin is administered as a continuous infusion to maintain a target activated clotting time (ACT) between 160 and 200 seconds. Other anticoagulants, such as bivalirudin or argatroban, may be used in patients with heparin-induced thrombocytopenia or heparin resistance.

• Monitoring anticoagulation: The medical team should monitor the patient's anticoagulation status closely to maintain the target ACT and prevent clot formation or bleeding complications. ACT should be measured at least every 4-6 hours, or more frequently if there are concerns about the patient's coagulation status.

- Bleeding complications: Anticoagulation increases the risk of bleeding complications, and the medical team should monitor the patient for signs of bleeding, such as hematomas, bleeding from puncture sites, or decreases in hemoglobin levels. The medical team should also minimize the use of invasive procedures and adjust anticoagulation as needed to prevent bleeding complications.

- Thrombotic complications: Despite anticoagulation, thrombotic complications can occur in some patients on ECMO therapy. The medical team should monitor the patient for signs of thrombosis, such as decreased ECMO flow or oxygenation, or evidence of clot formation in the ECMO circuit. In some cases, the medical team may need to increase anticoagulation or perform circuit changes to manage thrombotic complications.

- Monitoring platelets and coagulation factors: Anticoagulation can lead to depletion of platelets and coagulation factors, which can increase the risk of bleeding. The medical team should monitor the patient's platelet count, fibrinogen level, and other coagulation factors and adjust anticoagulation or administer blood products as needed to maintain adequate hemostasis.

- aPTT (Activated Partial Thromboplastin Time) is a laboratory test commonly used to monitor anticoagulation during ECMO (Extracorporeal Membrane Oxygenation) therapy. aPTT measures the time it takes for blood to clot in the presence of an activator and a phospholipid, and it is often used as a surrogate marker for heparin anticoagulation during ECMO therapy.

In summary, aPTT is a commonly used laboratory test to monitor anticoagulation during ECMO therapy. The medical team should monitor the patient's aPTT frequently and adjust heparin doses as needed to maintain optimal anticoagulation while minimizing the risk of bleeding or thrombotic complications.

Here are some key points about aPTT on ECMO:

1. Monitoring aPTT: aPTT should be monitored frequently in patients on ECMO therapy to assess the effectiveness of anticoagulation and to prevent both thrombotic and bleeding complications. aPTT is usually monitored every 4-6 hours, or more frequently if there are concerns about the patient's coagulation status.
2. Target range: The target range for aPTT during ECMO therapy varies depending on the patient's clinical condition, but aPTT is usually maintained between 1.5 and 2.5 times the patient's baseline value. However, the target aPTT may be adjusted based on the patient's bleeding or thrombotic risk.
3. Heparin dose adjustment: Heparin is the most commonly used anticoagulant during ECMO therapy, and heparin doses are adjusted based on the patient's aPTT levels. If the patient's aPTT is below the target range, the heparin dose may be increased, while if the aPTT is above the target range, the heparin dose may be decreased.
4. Other laboratory tests: In addition to aPTT, other laboratory tests such as platelet count, fibrinogen level, and antithrombin III level may be used to monitor the patient's coagulation status and adjust anticoagulation as needed.
5. Monitoring bleeding and thrombotic complications: Despite anticoagulation, bleeding and thrombotic complications can occur during ECMO therapy. The medical team should monitor the patient for signs of bleeding or thrombosis, such as hematomas, bleeding from puncture sites, or decreased oxygenation or ECMO flow, and adjust anticoagulation or perform circuit changes as needed.

Neurological Monitoring on ECMO

Patients who receive ECMO (Extracorporeal Membrane Oxygenation) therapy are at risk of neurological complications due to several factors, including underlying illness, hypoxemia, cerebral ischemia, and embolic events. Therefore, neurological monitoring is essential in patients receiving ECMO therapy to detect and manage any neurological complications promptly.

Here are some common methods of neurological monitoring for patients on ECMO:

1. Clinical examination: Clinical examination should be performed regularly to monitor neurological function, including the level of consciousness, pupillary response, motor function, and sensory function. Changes in neurological function should be reported to the medical team immediately.
2. Neuroimaging: Neuroimaging studies, such as computed tomography (CT) and magnetic resonance imaging (MRI), may be used to detect any neurological complications, such as ischemic or hemorrhagic stroke, and to monitor changes over time.
3. Continuous EEG (electroencephalography): Continuous EEG monitoring may be used to monitor for seizures or other abnormalities in brain function. It is particularly useful in patients at high risk of neurological complications, such as those with cardiac arrest or hypoxic-ischemic encephalopathy.
4. Transcranial Doppler (TCD): Transcranial Doppler is a non-invasive ultrasound technique that measures blood flow velocity in the cerebral vessels. TCD can be used to detect embolic events or changes in cerebral blood flow and can help guide management decisions.
5. Near-infrared spectroscopy (NIRS): NIRS is a non-invasive method that measures tissue oxygenation and perfusion in the brain. It can be used to monitor changes in cerebral oxygenation and to guide management decisions.

14. Ultrafiltration on ECMO

Ultrafiltration is a technique used during ECMO (Extracorporeal Membrane Oxygenation) therapy to remove excess fluid from the patient's blood. During this process, fluid can accumulate in the patient's body due to various factors, including inflammation, renal dysfunction, and increased capillary permeability.

Ultrafiltration can be performed by adding a filter to the ECMO circuit that removes excess fluid from the patient's blood, thus improving fluid balance and reducing the risk of complications such as pulmonary edema.

Here are some key points about ultrafiltration on ECMO:

1. Indications: Ultrafiltration may be indicated in patients on ECMO who have fluid overload, evidence of pulmonary edema, or worsening oxygenation despite other interventions.
2. Technique: Ultrafiltration involves adding a filter to the ECMO circuit that removes excess fluid from the patient's blood. The filter can be placed either before or after the oxygenator, and the ultrafiltrate is typically discarded.
3. Monitoring: The medical team should monitor the patient's fluid status closely during ultrafiltration, and adjust the ultrafiltration rate and volume based on the patient's response. Monitoring may include serial measurements of the patient's weight, urine output, and fluid balance.
4. Risks: Ultrafiltration may be associated with several risks, including hypotension, electrolyte imbalances, and bleeding. The medical team should closely monitor the patient's hemodynamic status and electrolyte levels during ultrafiltration, and adjust the ultrafiltration rate and volume as needed to minimize these risks.

Ultrafiltration can improve fluid balance and reduce the risk of complications such as pulmonary edema, but it should be performed with caution and close monitoring to minimize the risks of hypotension, electrolyte imbalances, and bleeding.

The connection of a hemofilter to the ECMO (Extracorporeal Membrane Oxygenation) circuit is an important step in performing ultrafiltration, a technique used to remove excess fluid from the patient's blood during ECMO therapy.

Here are the general steps for connecting a hemofilter to the ECMO circuit:

1. Select the appropriate hemofilter: The hemofilter should be selected based on the patient's size, blood flow rate, and ultrafiltration needs. The medical team should follow the manufacturer's instructions for use and ensure that the hemofilter is compatible with the ECMO circuit.
2. Prepare the hemofilter: The hemofilter should be primed with sterile saline or heparinized saline according to the manufacturer's instructions. The hemofilter should be checked for air bubbles and leaks before connecting it to the ECMO circuit.
3. Locate the appropriate port: The hemofilter can be connected to the ECMO circuit either before or after the oxygenator, depending on the medical team's preference. The medical team should locate the appropriate port on the ECMO circuit and ensure that the hemofilter is connected in the correct direction.
4. Connect the hemofilter: The hemofilter should be connected to the ECMO circuit using sterile technique. The medical team should follow the manufacturer's instructions for connecting the hemofilter, and ensure that all connections are secure and free from leaks.
5. Monitor the patient: The medical team should monitor the patient's fluid balance closely during ultrafiltration, and adjust the ultrafiltration rate and volume based on the patient's response. Monitoring may include serial measurements of the patient's weight, urine output, and fluid balance.
6. Disconnect the hemofilter: After completing ultrafiltration, the hemofilter should be disconnected from the ECMO circuit and disposed of according to the medical center's waste management policies.

15. Maintenance of ECMO circuit

Maintenance needs to be in place to ensure the pumps and other components are in perfect working order, and sufficient stocks of tubing, connectors and oxygenators are required.

An ECMO circuit can be primed with crystalloid fluids in advance of its use, as long as a strict aseptic technique is used. This circuit can be kept in a safe area for several weeks. The benefit of a primed circuit that is immediately available is obvious in case of sudden mechanical failure.

Failure is often not an option (back-up equipment must be available, as mechanical failure may happen even in perfectly maintained devices). Bespoke systems allow greater flexibility, as only the broken component (usually the pump motor) needs replacing.

Key points

- ECMO circuits should be as simple as possible.

- Modern centrifugal pumps are used in most systems. These are preload dependent and afterload sensitive.

- Monitoring of circuit pressures and blood flow is vital.

- Visual inspection is paramount to ensure circuit integrity.

ECMO circuit should be kept in sterile zone and under sterile conditions to avoid infections.

16. Clinical setup & Monitoring

PRIME :
 When Cardiac support is required, clear prime may be sufficient. In other cases prime with arterial blood and FFP, always add 800 IU heparin per unit of blood product, avoid NaHCO3 as buffer and prefer buffer agent TAM.

GOALS :
Hgb 12-15g/100 ml in neonate.
> 12 g/100 ml in Children & Adults

ANTICOAGULATION :
Initial dose 100 IU heparin/Kg IV.
Maintain with 15-16 IU/Kg/hr on syringe pump.
Recomended ACT between 150 to 180 sec when the circuit has a nontrombogenic surface.

ANTIBIOTICS :
According to institute protocol.

SEDATION :
Morphine 0.1 mg/Kg IV (Repeat as needed)

VASODIALATION :
Regitine (Phentolamine) 0.1-5.0 mg/Kg/min in neonates

VENTILATOR SETTING :
The ventilator is pressure controlled on ECMO

Neonates and Infants :
Reduce gradually to FiO2 - 0.3 (0.2 - 0.4)
over 1-2 hours if possible. Airway pressure 20/5 cm H_2O
Rate : 10/min
Peep : 4cm H_2O

Pediatrics & Adults :
FiO   0.4 - 0.5 . Peak airway pressure 20 - 30 cm H_2O
Rate : 10-15/min. Peep 10cm H_2O

Remark :

During Veno-arterial ECMO the patient will usually become alkalotic and the lungs may turn dense after the start of the ECMO.

Avoid rectum monitoring of temperature that may cause mucosal bleeding.

Negative pressure in venous line :
Pediatic 0-40mmHg
Adult 0-80mmHg

Monitor pressure before oxygenator inlet and after oxygenator outlet to check membrane function.

Daily Tests :

(LD, ASAT, ALAT, Hgb, BUN)
Electrolytes (K+ , Mg, Ca)
ACT for coagulation status
Hct, platelets, WBC

17. Weaning OFF ECMO

It's recommended to change the tube and rinse the airway before weaning from ECMO. The ECMO flow is reduced by 60-70% during 12-24 hours. Reduce the sweep gas to the oxygenatoruntil PCO2 is kept between 4-6kPa. Reduce FiO2 till 21. Increase the respiratory support to satisfactory O2 saturation.

Keep ACT > 200 seconds (180-250)

Stop the ECMO support to check the patient's response and ability to oxygenate and remove CO2 on its own.

Clamp the Arterial and Venous tubing.

keep the ECMO setup ready by recirculating the circuit to avoid coagulationof the system. If required the same setup can be used to support the patient till the patient is stable and ready for weaning from ECMO.

After weaning from ECMO discard the circuit with safety measures to avoid infection and blood spillag.

Initiating weaning from ECMO involves a systematic approach that considers the patient's condition, response to treatment, and readiness to have ECMO support reduced.

It is important to note that the weaning process should be individualized to each patient's specific condition and response to treatment. The healthcare team will closely monitor the patient throughout the weaning process and make adjustments as necessary to ensure the best possible outcome.

18. Cannula size selection for ECMO

The selection of cannula size for ECMO (Extracorporeal membrane oxygenation) is crucial for safe and effective treatment. The size of the cannula should be appropriate for the patient's weight and vascular anatomy to ensure adequate blood flow and minimize the risk of complications.

Here are some general guidelines for selecting cannula size for ECMO based on patient weight:

1. For neonates and infants weighing less than 10 kg, a 8-10 French (Fr) cannula is typically used for the arterial line, and a 12-14 Fr cannula is used for the venous line.
2. For infants and children weighing 10-25 kg, a 10-12 Fr cannula is typically used for the arterial line, and a 14-16 Fr cannula is used for the venous line.
3. For children and adolescents weighing 25-50 kg, a 12-14 Fr cannula is typically used for the arterial line, and a 18-20 Fr cannula is used for the venous line.
4. For adults weighing more than 50 kg, a 14-18 Fr cannula is typically used for the arterial line, and a 22-28 Fr cannula is used for the venous line.

It is important to note that these are general guidelines, and the selection of cannula size may need to be individualized based on the patient's vascular anatomy, medical history, and other factors.

Dear readers,

I want to express my heartfelt gratitude for your interest and support of the perfusion technology book that I have written. I am truly honored to have had the opportunity to share my knowledge and experience with you.
It is my sincere hope that the information presented in the book has been helpful in advancing your understanding of perfusion technology, and has provided practical guidance on the use of cardiopulmonary bypass and other essential techniques in cardiac surgery. I have worked hard to ensure that the book is comprehensive, up-to-date, and accessible to a wide range of healthcare professionals involved in perfusion technology.
Your feedback and engagement is crucial to the success of this book, and I am grateful for your support. I hope that it will continue to serve as a valuable resource for you, and that it will contribute to improving patient outcomes and advancing the field of cardiac surgery.

Once again, thank you for your interest in this book, and for your dedication to improving healthcare through the use of perfusion technology.

Sincerely,

Vivek .V. Paul
(Cardiac Perfusionist)

Made in the USA
Las Vegas, NV
04 December 2023

82106232R00024